Soiling in Child

About the Author

Prof. Alexander von Gontard, MD, is the director of the Department of Child and Adolescent Psychiatry, Saarland University Hospital, Germany, and holds the Chair for Child Psychiatry. He was trained in pediatrics, child psychiatry, and psychotherapy and has researched and published widely on incontinence in children and adolescents.

Soiling in Children and Adolescents

A Practical Guide for Parents, Teachers, and Caregivers

Alexander von Gontard
Department of Child and Adolescent Psychiatry,
Saarland University Hospital, Homburg, Germany

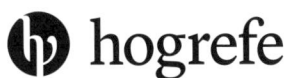

Library of Congress Cataloging in Publication information for the print version of this book is available via the Library of Congress Marc Database under the Library of Congress Control Number 2016930838

Library and Archives Canada Cataloguing in Publication Data

Gontard, Alexander von, author
  Soiling in children and adolescents : a practical guide for parents, teachers, and caregivers / Alexander von Gontard (Department of Child and Adolescent Psychiatry, Saarland University Hospital, Homburg, Germany).

Includes bibliographical references.
Issued in print and electronic formats.
ISBN 978-0-88937-487-4 (paperback).--ISBN 978-1-61676-487-6 (pdf).--ISBN 978-1-61334-487-3 (epub)

  1. Fecal incontinence in children. 2. Fecal incontinence in children--Treatment. 3. Urinary incontinence in children. 4. Urinary incontinence in children--Treatment. 5. Toilet training. I. Title.

RJ456.F43G65 2016   618.92'849   C2016-900284-5
                                           C2016-900285-3

This present volume is an adaptation and translation of A. von Gontard, *Ratgeber Einkoten* (2010, ISBN 978-3-801 2275-3), published under license from Hogrefe Verlag GmbH & Co. KG, Göttingen, Germany.
© 2010 by Hogrefe Verlag. Translated and revised by Alexander von Gontard, 2016.

The authors and publisher have made every effort to ensure that the information contained in this text is in accord with the current state of scientific knowledge, recommendations, and practice at the time of publication. In spite of this diligence, errors cannot be completely excluded. Also, due to changing regulations and continuing research, information may become outdated at any point. The authors and publisher disclaim any responsibility for any consequences which may follow from the use of information presented in this book.

Registered trademarks are not noted specifically in this publication. The omission of any such notice by no means implies that any trade names mentioned are free and unregistered.

The cover image is an agency photo depicting models. Use of the photo on this publication by no means implies any connection between the content of this publication and any person depicted in the cover image.

© 2017 by Hogrefe Publishing
http://www.hogrefe.com

PUBLISHING OFFICES

USA:	Hogrefe Publishing Corporation, 7 Bulfinch Place, 2nd floor, Boston, MA 02114
	Phone (866) 823-4726, Fax (617) 354-6875; E-mail customerservice@hogrefe.com
EUROPE:	Hogrefe Publishing GmbH, Merkelstr. 3, 37085 Göttingen, Germany
	Phone +49 551 99950-0, Fax +49 551 99950-111; E-mail publishing@hogrefe.com

SALES & DISTRIBUTION

USA:	Hogrefe Publishing, Customer Services Department,
	30 Amberwood Parkway, Ashland, OH 44805
	Phone (800) 228-3749, Fax (419) 281-6883; E-mail customerservice@hogrefe.com
UK:	Hogrefe Publishing, c/o Marston Book Services Ltd., 160 Eastern Ave.,
	Milton Park, Abingdon, OX14 4SB, UK
	Phone +44 1235 465577, Fax +44 1235 465556; E-mail direct.orders@marston.co.uk
EUROPE:	Hogrefe Publishing, Merkelstr. 3, 37085 Göttingen, Germany
	Phone +49 551 99950-0, Fax +49 551 99950-111; E-mail publishing@hogrefe.com

OTHER OFFICES

CANADA:	Hogrefe Publishing, 660 Eglinton Ave. East, Suite 119-514, Toronto, Ontario, M4G 2K2
SWITZERLAND:	Hogrefe Publishing, Länggass-Strasse 76, CH-3000 Bern 9

Hogrefe Publishing
Incorporated and registered in the Commonwealth of Massachusetts, USA, and in Göttingen, Lower Saxony, Germany

No part of this book may be reproduced, stored in a retrieval system or transmitted, in any form or by any means, electronic, mechanical, photocopying, microfilming, recording or otherwise, without written permission from the publisher.

Cover image: © Aldo Murillo – istockphoto.com

Printed and bound in Germany

ISBN 978-0-88937-487-4 (print) • ISBN 978-1-61676-487-6 (PDF) • ISBN 978-1-61334-487-3 (EPUB)
http://doi.org/10.1027/00487-000

Table of Contents

Aims of this guide 1

How should I use this guide? 3

1 General Information on Soiling 5
1.1 Does this sound familiar to you? 5
1.2 What is the definition of soiling? 7
1.3 What types of soiling are there? 10
1.4 How common is soiling? 12
1.5 What are the causes of soiling? 12
1.6 If common prejudices about soiling are not true, how can soiling be explained? 14
1.7 Could my soiling child have a psychological problem? 16
1.8 Why does my child also wet? 17
1.9 Which examinations are needed for the assessment of soiling? 18
1.10 How should soiling be treated? 22

2 Soiling With Constipation 24
2.1 How do you recognize soiling with constipation? 24
2.2 How does soiling with constipation develop? 26
2.3 How do you treat soiling with constipation? 29
2.4 When are laxatives necessary? 31
2.5 How is disimpaction performed? 32

2.6	What happens during the maintenance phase?	35
2.7	What is toilet training?	38
2.8	What to do if treatment fails?	42
2.9	What can I do if my child has special needs?	43
3	**Soiling Without Constipation**	45
3.1	What is soiling without constipation?	45
3.2	How do you treat soiling without constipation?	46
4	**Toilet Refusal**	48
4.1	How does toilet refusal develop?	48
4.2	How do you treat toilet refusal?	49
5	**Soiling With Wetting**	52
5.1	How does soiling with wetting develop?	52
5.2	What is the definition of daytime wetting?	53
5.3	What is bedwetting?	55
5.4	How is wetting assessed?	56
5.5	How do you treat daytime wetting?	56
5.6	How do you treat bedwetting?	59
5.7	How do you treat combined soiling and wetting?	62
6	**Soiling and Psychological Problems**	64
6.1	How common are psychological problems and disorders in children who soil?	64
6.2	How do you assess psychological disorders?	66

| 6.3 | How do you treat soiling if psychological problems or disorders are present? | 66 |
| 6.4 | Where can you treat soiling and psychological disorders? | 68 |

7 Concluding Remarks 70

Further Reading 71

Appendices 73
Appendix 1: Soiling Questionnaire 74
Appendix 2: 48-Hour Toilet Chart 76
Appendix 3: Drinking Chart 78
Appendix 4: Toilet Training Chart for Parents 79
Appendix 5: Toilet Training Chart for Children ... 80

Aims of this guide

The aim of this guide is to provide information on the different types of soiling and their causes as well as on how to assess and treat them effectively. The information is intended mainly for parents but may be useful for teachers, educators, caregivers, as well as older children and adolescents. The objective of this guide is to give short and precise advice on the most important forms of soling that might affect children and adolescents. While dealing with wetting problems has become acceptable in many countries, soiling is often still stigmatized. The distress in families is higher and children with soiling have far more psychological problems than those who wet. This guide provides practical advice, step-by-step instructions, and concrete recommendations on how to achieve continence. To make it more understandable, everyday terms such as *soiling*, *daytime wetting*, and *bedwetting* are used throughout the book instead of the scientific terms. Please feel free to copy the charts and materials included in the appendix and use them for your child.

This guide was first published in 2010 and has received positive feedback from many parents. As there are no comparable guidebooks in the English language, the time had come to make this information available for parents all over the world. Due to the many new developments, the book was not just translated but was brought up to date with many innovative aspects. All recommendations are based on current scientific studies and international guidelines. We considered both European and North American practice parameters and specifically followed the recommendations of the International Children's Continence Society (ICCS). The ICCS is a multi-professional, international organization that has set out to standardize the treatment of incontinence in children based on the newest scientific evidence. Following ICCS recommendations is the best way to ensure the welfare of children being treated for incontinence.

As many children not only soil but are also affected by wetting, a separate companion guide is available for this type of incontinence (*Wetting in children and adolescents: A practical guide for parents, teachers, and caregivers*; Hogrefe Publishing, 2017).

I would like to thank Hogrefe, and especially Mr. Robert Dimbleby and Ms. Juliane Munson, for their enthusiasm and support of this project. I hope very much that this guide will be of help to many families to achieve continence.

Saarbrücken, Germany, June 2016

Alexander von Gontard

How should I use this guide?

The aim of this guide is to provide the reader with information that is organized as logically and explained as simply as possible. The two most common forms of soiling, with and without constipation, are discussed right at the beginning before we talk about toilet refusal, soiling with wetting, and soiling in combination with psychological problems.

Soiling with constipation is the topic of Chapter 2. Basic aspects of treatment, which apply to all types of soiling, will be presented here.

Chapter 3 deals with soiling without constipation. Please also read Chapter 2 because the treatment basics for soiling with constipation are the same.

In Chapter 4, aspects of toilet refusal will be presented. This is relevant for children who insist on using the diaper for their bowel movements but do void urine into the toilet. If your child does not show this kind of behavior, you can skip this chapter.

Combined wetting and soiling is dealt with in Chapter 5. If your child does not wet, you can skip this chapter.

Chapter 6 is dedicated to the combination of soiling and psychological problems and disorders. If you do not see major problems in your child's behavior and emotional well-being, you can skip this chapter.

The aim of this guide is to provide you with practical information on soiling and ways to treat it. However, it is important that you seek professional help. Because medical causes of soiling have to be identified – or ruled out – before treatment can begin, every child or adolescent needs to be examined by a pediatrician or general practitioner. For a good assessment it can be of great help to fill out the Soiling Questionnaire (Appendix 1) before consulting your physician. If your child is affected by both soiling and wetting, the information collected in the 48-Hour Toilet Chart (Appendix 2) is of great importance. During treatment of soiling we recommend that you use the charts in Appendices 3, 4, and 5 as they can be very motivating and support the treatment. Please discuss the charts and any questions you might have with your physician or therapist.

We hope that you and your child will find this guide helpful and that you will reach continence quickly so that you can put this little book aside – or recommend it to friends.

1 General Information on Soiling

1.1 Does this sound familiar to you?

My daughter soils. In the afternoon, when she returns from school I know exactly what is going to happen. It may be during lunchtime, while doing homework, or at the very latest when she's playing. Sometimes the pants are just smeared, sometimes there are large amounts of stool in them. Sometimes my daughter seems to be distressed, but usually she seems not to care at all. She simply continues to play and does not go to the toilet until the underpants are completely full of poo. I feel completely helpless because I do not know what I've done wrong. I would like to help my daughter, but I do not know how. All the advice I have received so far has not helped. On some days, I am really angry, especially if I find hidden underpants full of feces. The stinky laundry is really not very pleasant. I simply wish that this would stop.

In contrast to other problems, many parents are often left alone with this plight. They often do not dare to even speak about it with other parents because other children seem to function so much better and are so successful – only their child seems to have these problems.

Many parents seek advice from their pediatrician, general practitioner, or therapist. When the soiling does not stop, parents sometimes seek psychotherapy or consult alternative medicine practitioners. This is a pity because effective treatments are available! The main requirement is that a good and careful assessment is performed, as different forms of soiling exist. Also, soiling may be – but does not need to be – combined with wetting as well as psychological problems and disorders. These two examples of Paul and Lisa illustrate the different types of soiling:

> Paul is a seven-year-old boy who has good grades in school. He is in second grade. Unfortunately, he disrupts class very often, he teases other children and does not follow the rules. Soiling never happens during school time but in the afternoons and evenings. Sometimes Paul soils large amounts of stool, which are either very hard or very liquid. Paul seldom goes to the toilet to move his bowels. Sometimes 2 or 3 days will pass before he goes to the toilet again. Moving his bowels is often very painful for him, and Paul often complains about tummy aches. He is a very picky eater and does not drink very much. Although he has been dry before, he began to wet his bed again when entering school. During the day, he doesn't go to the toilet very often to pee and his pants are nearly always wet. Paul is a very lively boy and often gets into long discussions and arguments when he is asked to do something.

> Lisa is in first grade and, just like Paul, never soils during school time. Although she has regular bowel movements every day, with her stool normally formed, she soils in the afternoons. She is very ashamed of the soiling and

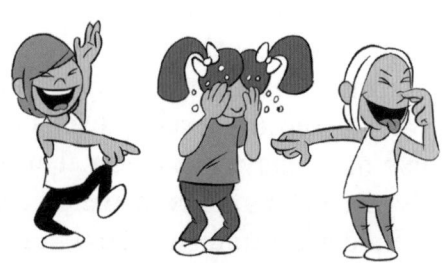

tries to hide it. She has been teased by her girlfriends and has cried bitterly. Apart from that, she has many interests and is socially well-integrated.

Do these or similar descriptions sound familiar to you? If yes, then this guide will be able to help you. Despite all the stress and worries induced by soiling, there is a very positive general message: Most children can become continent. Some children are very quick about it, while others need longer to overcome the problem. If parents and children cooperate actively, all efforts are well invested. Once children become continent, their self-confidence and feelings of self-worth increase – they feel happier and relaxed. At the same time, stress, tension, and worries in the families become less. The aim of this guide is to give you direct and practical suggestions on how to achieve this goal, step by step. But first, we will give you some general information.

1.2 What is the definition of soiling?

The scientific term for soiling is *encopresis*. Some specialists prefer the neutral term *fecal incontinence*. For easier understanding we will use the everyday term *soiling* throughout this book. Soiling is defined as repeated passing of bowels in inappropriate places from the age of four years onwards – after medical causes have been excluded. The most important aspects of soiling are reflected in this short definition. If a child soils once every few months, this is certainly not a reason to worry. Only if a child soils at least once a month for the duration of three months, the soiling is considered to be a real disorder or condition. If it occurs less than once a month, it can be a stressful experience but it is considered to be a temporary problem. If soiling happens to your child on rare occasions, try not to make a big fuss about it but comfort your child. Temporary soiling really does happen to many children.

Soiling can only be considered a disorder or condition when the child has reached his or her 4th birthday. Why is this age definition so important? The reason is that soiling is so common among three-year-old children that it is seen as part of natural maturation and not as a disorder.

The age range in the development of continence is enormous and varies greatly from child to child. Some children want to become continent as early as during their second year of life. They send out active signals that they would like to be potty trained. This initiative of the child can be encouraged by parents in a playful manner. If the child achieves continence, this is a huge developmental milestone and most children are extremely proud. Other children need more time – and this is completely normal, too. According to many studies, it is fine to grant two- and three-year-old children more time, giving them diapers if they wish, and to wait until their fourth birthday. Only from this age onwards, soiling is no longer seen as part of normal development but as a disorder that can be assessed and treated.

It is not important when potty training is started, but that parents support their child when he or she gives signals of being ready for training. Some children do this quite early, while others need more time. In contrast, potty training first and primarily started by parental prompting is not optimal. A few decades ago, when washing machines and throwaway diapers were not available, many parents tried to potty train their children at a very early age. Some even started potty training during infancy (during their first year of life) when a child is developmentally not able to control bladder and bowels. Nowadays, starting training too late is a more prevalent problem than early potty training. Some parents try not to put pressure on their children and support a laissez-faire attitude. They can sometimes overlook the signals their child gives or are afraid to prompt them. As a consequence, potty training is not supported by parents actively and is started too late. This, too, is not optimal for children.

In addition to age of potty training, the tone and atmosphere in which it is conducted is decisive. A pleasant and playful atmosphere makes it much easier for the child to gain bowel control – and the joy is great when this has been achieved. Pressure, threats, shouting, or punishment will not lead to earlier continence – to the contrary, the likelihood for soiling at a later point increases greatly. Similarly, little interest in or support for potty training will also not be helpful.

All in all, the definitional age of four years makes a lot of sense. Parents should give their child all the time he or she needs – and support their child actively when he or she is ready to be potty trained. They should not be discouraged or unsettled by preschool teachers. In some countries, prejudices abound that every child has to be continent before entering preschool. This is simply not true and not very considerate of the individual development of the child. It is not a problem for a child to go to preschool wearing a diaper. If the diaper needs to be changed, teachers can assist the child. Also don't let friends or relatives upset or unsettle you – your child does have time to become continent until he or she is four years old.

1.3 What types of soiling are there?

Soiling occurs almost exclusively during the day. If it does happen during the night, this should be a reason to be especially careful with medical examinations, as nighttime soiling is more often due to a somatic or medical cause. The usual presentation of soiling is during the day.

In the past, soiling was differentiated into primary and secondary soiling. Primary means that the child has never been continent for more than six months in a row. In contrast, secondary soiling designates a relapse after the child has been continent for at least six consecutive months. Since recent studies have shown that there are no differences between primary and secondary soiling and because treatment is the same for both types, the differentiation into primary and secondary soiling has no practical relevance for assessment and treatment and is no longer needed.

The most important question that you have to answer is: Does your child just soil – or is he or she also constipated? Finding out whether the child is constipated is the most important step for treatment, but constipation is not always easy to detect. It is not sufficient to note how often

1. General Information on Soiling

a child goes to the bathroom. For children who go to the toilet only once or twice per week it seems obvious and constipation can be suspected. Other children pass their bowels every day on the toilet but still hold back stool and are constipated. They often feel pain when they have bowel movements as stool can be very hard. When the abdomen is felt with the hands, one can even detect the hard stool masses, which are also visible in ultrasound examination. Here, soiling is a consequence of constipation and retention of stool. Abdominal pains and reduced appetite are also common for these children. The most common type of constipation is *functional constipation*, i.e., when medical causes have been ruled out.

Other children soil but are not constipated at all. This type of constipation is called *nonretentive fecal incontinence*. In this case, it is much more difficult to understand why the children soil. But no matter what the causes of soiling are, effective ways of treating the children are always available.

Some children pass urine when on the toilet but stubbornly refuse to move their bowels. They demand to have a diaper for their bowel movements. This behavior, which worries many parents, is called *toilet refusal*. It is completely harmless if it persists for only a short time. If toilet refusal, however, continues for months or even years, constipation is likely to develop.

You will hear more about the different types of soiling in later chapters.

1.4 How common is soiling?

Many parents are astonished to hear how common soiling actually is among children. They are often convinced that only their child is affected by this problem. And yet, soiling is one of the most common disorders of childhood. Between age 4 and 16, 1–3 % of all children and adolescents are affected, which comes out to a large number of children. Three groups of children with different soiling behavior can be identified. Some children continue to soil continuously over many years. Others have times when they are continent – and times when they relapse. In the third group, the rate and likelihood of soiling slowly diminishes over time in the process of natural maturation.

The prevalence of soiling is lower during late adolescence, but studies and exact figures are not yet available. We do know, however, that if soiling is not treated for a sufficiently long time during childhood, it can persist into adolescence and even young adulthood. It can turn into a chronic condition children and adolescents may not grow out of. Therefore, "waiting it out" is not the way to go. Early and intensive treatment of soiling is a good start for long-term success.

1.5 What are the causes of soiling?

This question is a real concern for many parents and children. Unfortunately, lack of information and prejudices are common, not just in families but also among teachers, therapists, and even physicians.

A common prejudice among less informed preschool teachers is that a child who soils is simply not developmentally mature. It does happen that a child with soiling is not allowed to enter preschool – sometimes preschool teachers even refuse to assist in changing diapers. As mentioned previously, every child has its own developmental pace – some are quicker, others are slower. Soiling is not a sign of maturational delay.

Another misconception is that parents could cause the soiling of their child. Therefore, many parents worry and wonder what they have possibly done wrong. Recent studies have shown that most parents of children who soil are very worried about them, are distressed themselves, and want to do everything they can to help their children stop soiling. Placing blame or feeling guilty is never helpful for a successful treatment. It is also not very useful to ruminate about the past. Instead, parents should look ahead and actively start treatment with their children!

As discussed in Chapter 1.2, early and child-initiated potty training might lead to earlier continence in individual children (and save a lot of diapers and washing). Studies have also shown that early potty training does not reduce – or increase – the rate of soiling at age 4 (the definitional age for a disorder). In contrast, late potty training has been shown to be associated with toilet refusal, constipation, and soiling.

Another common idea is that soiling is a purely psychological condition. This opinion is still voiced by many psychotherapists, although it is completely obsolete. Many studies have shown that approximately 30–50% of all children with soiling have manifest behavioral problems or disorders. There is a wide range of possible disorders: Some children are depressed and anxious while others are hyperactive and do not follow rules and are disobedient. No specific disorder is typical for soiling or could be the exclusive explanation for the problem. If your child soils and does have additional psychological problems, then both issues should be addressed and treated. The treatment of soiling always has priority.

Looking at the figures the other way around, you can see that 50–70% of children soil without having psychological symptoms or a disorder. In these cases, of course, only the soiling is treated. Psychotherapy is not indicated and should be avoided. It is not effective and can even delay continence.

1.6 If common prejudices about soiling are not true, how can soiling be explained?

Two general aspects are important if one is looking for causes:
- First, there is usually not one single cause but several different causes which are connected with each other. In many cases, it is not possible to find a single definite cause for soiling.
- Second, it is really not important to know the exact causes. Many parents think or hope that the problem will be solved as soon as the cause has been found. Usually, the opposite is true: The identification of causes will not suddenly stop the soiling, and it is not necessary to know them for sucessful treatment. There-

fore, it is much more important for parents to concentrate on the present and the future and to dedicate themselves to active treatment.

The reasons for the development of **soiling with constipation** are well researched. Genetic disposition plays an important role in constipation. Chronic constipation develops out of acute constipation, which is quite common in infants and toddlers. Acute constipation can be triggered by a variety of events, for example, by pain experienced during bowel movement due to painful fissures in the anal region. Also, stressful life events like moving home, the separation of parents, or the birth of a sibling can act as triggers. The child begins to hold back stool, the gut enlarges, and a vicious circle develops causing more and more stool masses to be retained. Soiling then develops as a consequence of the constipation. This form of soiling will be dealt with in more detail in Chapter 2.

Causative associations are not well known for children who soil without constipation. We do not know exactly why children who do not have problems with stool retention soil, but genetic factors seem to play a less important role in this type of soiling. **Soiling without constipation** is certainly not a purely psychological condition, as many recent studies have shown. The rate of co-occurring psychological problems and disorders is approximately the same for both types of soiling (approx. 30–50% of all children are affected) – irrespective of constipation being present or not. More information on soiling without constipation will be presented in Chapter 3.

If children show **toilet refusal** for only a short time, it may just be a temporary habit. In chronic toilet refusal, constipation can develop as an additional risk factor. Some of these children show oppositional defiant behavior or have other psychological problems. You can read more about the interactions of soiling and behavioral problems in Chapter 4.

1.7 Could my soiling child have a psychological problem?

This is a question that worries many parents. As mentioned above, most soiling children do not have behavioral problems. For these children soiling is a chronic and automatic habit that is maintained despite its disadvantages. It is absolutely sufficient to treat the soiling alone to achieve continence. But even if children are distressed, anxious, or sad, treatment of the soiling may be all they need. When they have reached continence, distressful worries disappear, self-confidence rises, and children feel relieved and relaxed.

Between 30 and 50% of children with soiling have additional, clinically relevant disorders, which can lead to additional impairments. Several types of disorders can be observed. Some children suffer from depression or anxiety disorders (so-called *internalizing disorders*); others have attention-deficit/hyperactivity disorder (ADHD), oppositional defiant disorder (ODD), or even conduct disorders (so-called *externalizing disorders*). Exact assessment of soiling and the other problems is necessary. Soiling should always be treated. ADHD, anxiety and other disorders have to be treated as well because they will not disappear of their own accord. In addition, children with ADHD are known to be less cooperative and adhere less to therapy so that soiling could persist for a longer time if ADHD is not treated.

In some cases, all present disorders (i.e., soiling and behavioral issues) can be treated simultaneously. Sometimes, however, it may be more appropriate to treat one problem after the other. Whatever the case, ask the advice of your pediatrician, general practitioner, child psychiatrist, or child psychologist who will help you plan the treatment. Please refer to Chapter 6 for more information about soiling and psychological problems.

1.8 Why does my child also wet?

This is another question that many parents ask themselves. Combined soiling and wetting is so typical that an official term has been created for it: *bowel and bladder dysfunction* (BDD). Most children wet during the day, some during the night, and some even days and nights. Again, exact assessment is necessary. Clear and established recommendations for the treatment sequence are available: Soiling is always treated first because some children stop wetting when soiling and constipation have been tackled successfully. Daytime wetting should be treated before nighttime wetting because bedwetting is likely to stop once the daytime problems have been solved. If your child continues to wet during the night, this can be treated well at the end. You will find detailed information about soiling and wetting in Chapter 5.

1.9 Which examinations are needed for the assessment of soiling?

Because of possible medical causes and complications, each child should be examined by a pediatrician or general practitioner at least once. If your child is constipated, medical causes are likely in up to 5% of all cases. The rate of somatic causes in children without constipation is much lower, i.e., less than 1% of all cases. Only if medical and somatic causes have been excluded, can soiling be diagnosed as a condition called encopresis or fecal incontinence. Part of the definition of encopresis or fecal incontinence is that there are no medical causes – it is a purely functional disorder. The good news is, of course, that functional disorders can be reversed and cured.

Usually, a simple physical examination by your doctor is sufficient. More detailed examinations are only necessary if a medical condition is suspected. Try to avoid all unnecessary, especially invasive, examinations for your child – because he or she probably won't need them.

The following standard assessment program is enough for the majority of children with soiling problems:
1. A detailed history of soiling, of previous treatments, and of the development of your child is the first step of assessment.
2. In addition, questionnaires regarding soiling problems have proven to be very useful. The information gathered by the Soiling Questionnaire (see Appendix 1) is important for planning optimal treatment for your child. Going through this questionnaire might also help you understand the soiling and toileting behavior of

your child. The Bristol Stool Form Scale (see Figure 1) has proven to be useful for the assessment of stool consistency – both for feces passed on the toilet and during soiling incidents. Numbers 3–5 designate normal types of stool while the other types are more common in constipation and soiling. Please let your pediatrician or general practitioner know which type of stool consistency is typical for when your child soils and when he or she passes stool on the toilet.

3. Since 30–50% of all children with soiling have additional behavioral problems, it is important to assess whether a disorder is present or not. The type of disorder should be diagnosed as this has direct consequences for treatment. For children without behavioral problems, the treatment of soiling is sufficient. Should other problems be diagnosed, then these have to be treated in addition to the soiling. Therefore, it is recommended that a validated, broadband behavioral questionnaire is filled out by all parents. Examples are the internationally established Child Behavior Checklist (CBCL) or the Strengths and Difficulties Questionnaire (SDQ). The CBCL is distributed commercially while the SDQ can be downloaded for free at http://www.sdqinfo.com. If you like, complete the questionnaires and show them to your pediatrician or general practitioner. If you and your doctor notice that many problem items are checked on these questionnaires, a mental health care assessment by a child psychologist or psychiatrist is advisable. If a disorder is present, counseling and treatment can be extremely helpful, reduce distress, and increase your child's ability to cooperate with soiling treatment.

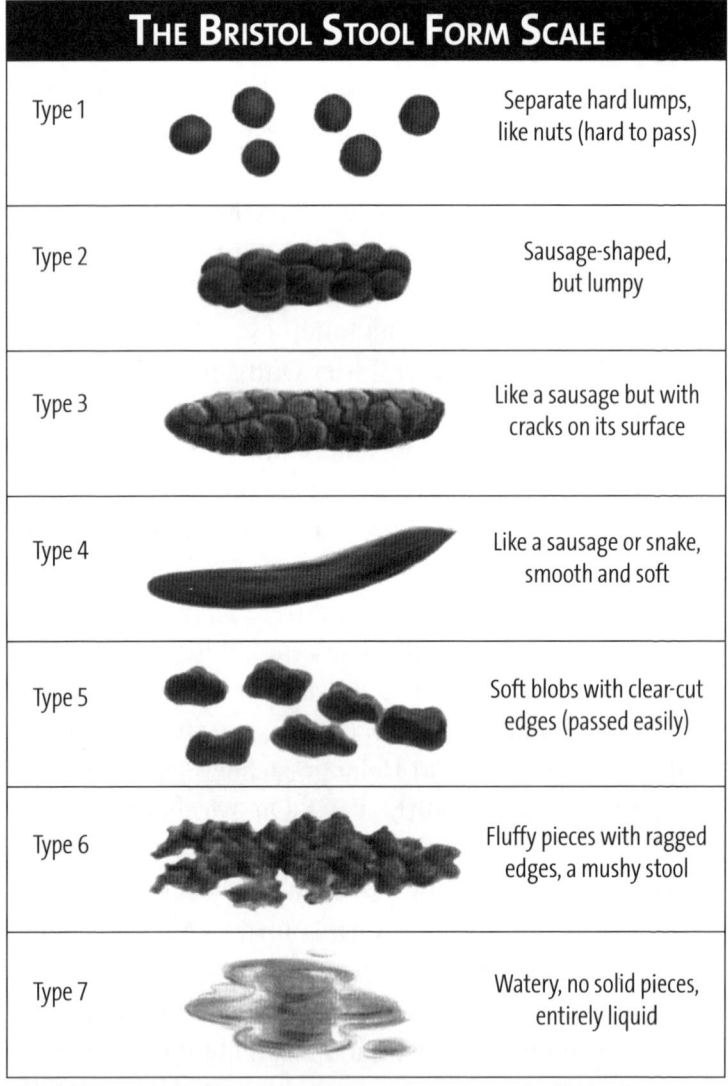

Figure 1. Bristol Stool Form Scale. Types 3–5 are considered normal. The other types are typical for constipation and soiling.

4. As mentioned previously, your child should be examined by a physician at least once at the beginning of treatment. The back, genital, and anal area should always be looked at to rule out anomalies.
5. One ultrasound examination of the abdomen, rectum, bladder, and kidneys is recommended. Measuring the diameter of the rectum is an important part of assessment. The rectum can easily be observed as round or oval shape behind the bladder. If the diameter is greater than 30 mm ($\approx$ 1 inch), it is likely that your child is retaining stool masses. In soiling without constipation, the diameter is usually less than 30 mm. Also, ultrasound can be very helpful to monitor the effects of laxative treatment as one can see directly how the diameter of the rectum decreases. This can be very motivating for parents and children.
6. If your child wets and soils, the completion of the 48-Hour Toilet Chart is recommended (see Appendix 2). Parents are asked to note down the drinking and toileting behavior of their child on two consecutive days, for example, on weekends when there are no other obligations or stress factors present. The time and amount of drinking fluids should be noted as many children with soiling do not drink sufficient amounts. The amount of urine should be measured with a measuring cup and written down in the chart – as should all incidents of soiling and wetting as well as bowel movements on the toilet. The last column is used to note down any other observations, such as holding maneuvers (pressing the thighs together, jumping from one foot to the next, or holding the tummy).

7. A urine analysis with the help of a test strip (drip stick) to exclude the presence of a urinary tract infection is recommended for children who wet and soil.

This standard assessment is really all that most children with soiling need. Other examinations should only be carried out if other medical conditions are suspected. Your physician will be able to advise you. If your child does need more specialized assessment and care, it is extremely important that this is carried out by specialists, such as pediatric gastroenterologists (specialized in stomach and intestinal problems) or pediatric surgeons who are well informed about childhood disorders. In some countries, children are admitted to hospitals for adults – this is a practice we do not recommend. There is great danger that unnecessary examinations are carried out. Therefore, it is very important that you consult only pediatric specialists if this is needed.

1.10 How should soiling be treated?

In this section you will find general recommendations. More detailed information will be given in later chapters.
1. The detailed assessment by a physician or other practitioner should always be the first step of treatment. Do not start treatment before your child has been examined. This is necessary to exclude medical causes or other complications and to diagnose the type of soiling and possible associated behavioral disorders.
2. Ineffective methods should be discontinued. Some parents try alternative, herbal, or homeopathic methods which generally do not work. Because sometimes in-

effective medication that can even be harmful is prescribed, it is a good idea to stop all unnecessary methods of treatment.
3. You should insist that information on soiling is presented to you in an understandable way. Only if you and your child understand all aspects, will you be convinced and motivated to start and continue treatment. Please feel free to ask all the questions that you have.
4. The basic treatment approach for both types of soiling is the same and consists of intensive toilet training (see Chapter 2.7). This has to be carried out regularly and over a longer period of time.
5. Only if your child is constipated, it is necessary to use laxatives (see Chapter 2.5). At the beginning of treatment, all retained stool masses have to be evacuated. This is called *disimpaction* (see Chapter 2.5). Once the stool has been passed, the aim is to avoid re-accumulation by carrying out toilet training and using oral laxatives. It is very important that both toilet training and laxatives are continued for long enough, sometimes for months or even years.
6. If your child soils but is not constipated, laxatives should never be given as they can worsen the soiling (see Chapter 3).
7. In combined soiling and wetting, the established sequence of treatment is: soiling first, followed by daytime wetting and, finally, bedwetting (see Chapter 5).
8. If your child has additional behavioral problems or disorders, these have to be treated separately (see Chapter 6). While this is ongoing, the basic treatment of soiling should be continued (i.e., toilet training and, if indicated, laxatives).

2 Soiling With Constipation

The most important types of soiling are soiling with constipation and soiling without constipation. Functional constipation, i.e., constipation not due to medical causes, is a common problem worldwide and affects many children. The exact prevalence of constipation is not known because different definitions are used and constipation can easily be overlooked by physicians.

However, constipation is more common than soiling. Between 70 and 90% of children with constipation also soil. Between 50 and 70% of children who soil are also constipated. This means that soiling with constipation is more common than the second type, soiling without constipation.

2.1 How do you recognize soiling with constipation?

Not long ago, people used to think that constipation can be recognized easily. If children rarely went to the toilet to move their bowels, this was seen as the main sign of constipation. Studies have shown that starting at age 4, most children have bowel movements once a day – with great variation from child to child. If children had three or fewer bowel movements per week, i.e.,

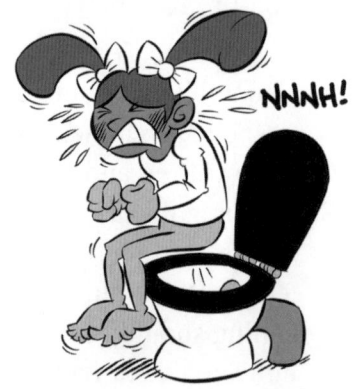

fewer than one every other day, they were considered to be constipated.

We know by now that things are more complicated than that. Some children retain stool continuously even though they go to the toilet every day to move their bowels – they are still constipated. Therefore, it is important to watch out for other signs of constipation. One typical sign is that the stool passed on the toilet is very hard. Because the diameter of the rectum may be enlarged, the amounts of passed stool can be enormous. When the children soil, the stool is either hard or soft, but it is usually not well formed (see the Bristol Stool Form Scale in Figure 1). Many children complain about pain when their stool is hard. They also often complain about general tummy aches. Their appetite may be reduced and they are often picky eaters. Many parents overlook the fact that their children do not drink enough, which is very common among children who soil. Physicians can feel the built-up stool, called *skybalous masses*, through the abdomen. The rectum, which is often enlarged, is visible in ultrasound examinations. The rectum diameter is considered to be larger than normal when it is above 30 mm (≈ 1 inch). This is very typical in constipation.

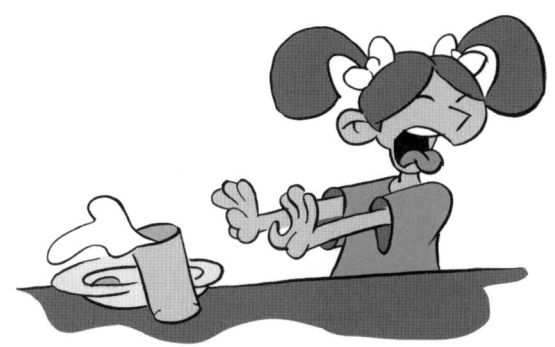

Taking these individual symptoms together, the diagnosis of constipation is clear. Knowing that the child is constipated is important for the planning of the entire treatment.

As mentioned in Chapter 1, the diagnosis soiling means that it occurs over at least three consecutive months with a frequency of at least one soiling incident per month. For the diagnosis of soiling it is not relevant to know whether the pants are just smeared or whether there are large amounts of stool. The aim of treatment is complete continence and not just the reduction of the soiled amount of stool.

2.2 How does soiling with constipation develop?

Again, not one but several factors play a role in the development of constipation. Genetic predisposition may be a factor because constipation runs in families. Parents and siblings are also often constipated; fathers and brothers are especially affected. In twin studies it was observed that identical twins are both more affected than fraternal twins. If one parent has constipation, the risk for the child to be constipated is 26%. If both parents are constipated, this risk increases to 50%.

Genetic factors are, of course, not the sole cause of constipation. Other environmental factors are needed to turn the predisposition into a condition. Triggers for constipation are common and varied. Very often *acute constipation* is caused when the child experiences pain during bowel movements because of fissures in the anal region, for example. They hold back stool in an effort to avoid the pain. Acute constipation can also start when new foods are introduced, for example, when changing from milk formula to solid food during infancy. Stressful life events, such as the separation or divorce of parents, moving home, the birth of siblings, entering kindergarten or school, and psychological factors, are common triggers of acute constipation. Usually, acute constipation is nothing to worry about because it does not last and ends without having further consequences. However, for some children acute constipation may start a vicious circle and lead to *chronic constipation*. Children continue to avoid moving their bowels and hold back hard stool. Parents are often familiar with the holding maneuvers of their children: They hop from one foot to the other as if they're dancing, hold their tummy, cross their legs, or sit on their heel.

Through the retention of stool, stool masses accumulate in the colon and rectum, i.e., the large intestine. This process is illustrated in Figure 2. The colon gets bigger while at the same time the ability to feel that the colon is full decreases. Most children, therefore, don't even notice that they have so much stool in their colon. In addition, the propulsion of the stool, i.e., the forward movement in the intestines, is reduced so that the stool is no longer transported quickly but remains in one place for a long time. Many studies have shown that the so-called *colon transit time*, i.e., the time it takes for food to be transported through the colon, is much longer in children with constipation. Because of the increased time in the colon a lot of fluid is drawn from the stool. It gets hard and forms big, solid lumps that are almost like rocks. These lumps stay in the colon while new and more liquid stool passes

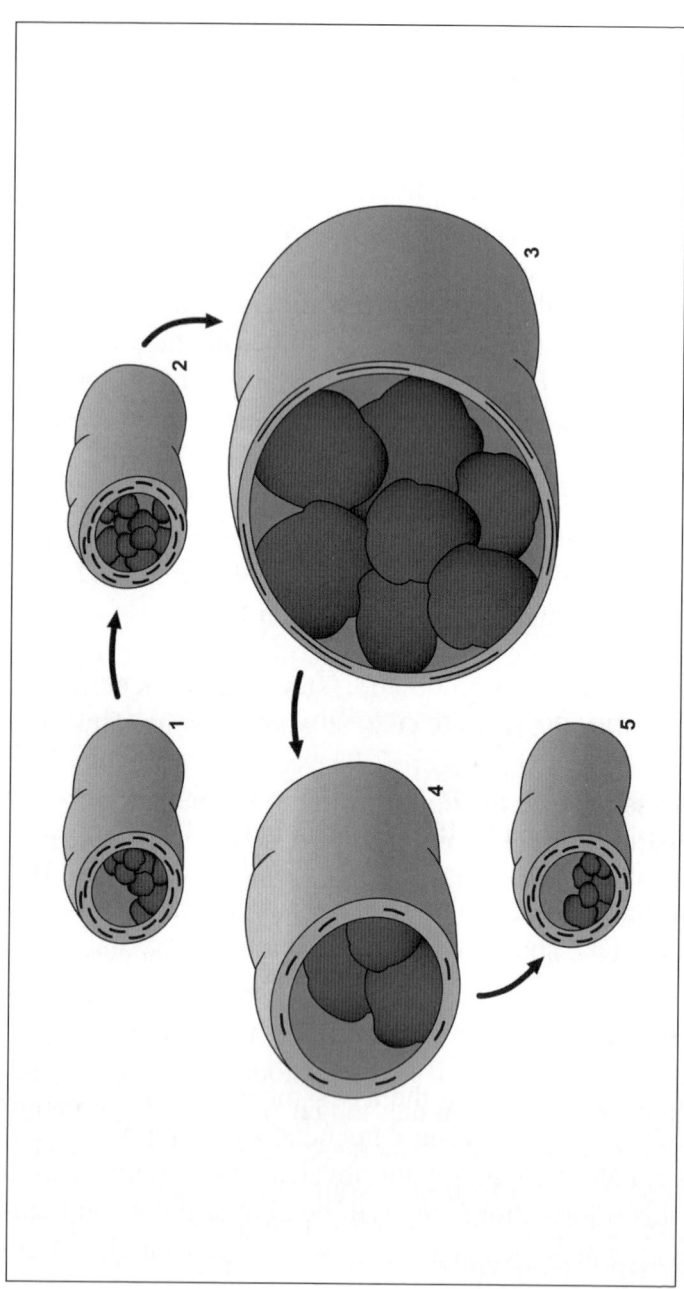

Figure 2. The development of constipation (1–3) and its resolution.

by and leaks into the pants, thus leading to soiling even though the child is constipated. The outdated term *overflow incontinence* tried to describe this phenomenon but it is not correct because stool does not overflow. Instead, a term like *in-between flow incontinence* would be more suitable. The older stool remains in the colon while fresh stool flows in between the lumps and leaks out.

Pictures 1–3 in Figure 2 show the build-up of constipation. Pictures 4 and 5 show the return of the colon to normal size under treatment.

If stool remains in the colon over weeks, months, or even years, the colon can grow to a very large size. An enlarged colon is visible in ultrasound and can be felt by your physician when examining the belly.

2.3 How do you treat soiling with constipation?

The first step of every treatment is the detailed assessment of the problem. It has to be confirmed that both soiling and constipation are present. Medical causes as well as psychological problems and disorders have to be excluded. One should take enough time for the diagnostic process because only a clear diagnosis will make successful treatment possible.

You can contribute to the assessment process by filling out the questionnaire in Appendix 1 (Soiling Questionnaire) before going to your physician or therapist. Based on this information, they will be able to tailor the treatment towards the needs of your child. If your child both soils and wets, be sure to also complete the 48-Hour Toilet Chart in Appendix 2. Especially the drinking behavior of your child is important for your physician to know.

Proper counseling and good information are essential for parents and children at the beginning of treatment. Many parents and children do not realize that the retention of stool in combination with constipation is the main cause of the soiling. Some believe that the anus does not close properly and, therefore, causes stool to leak out and are surprised to learn that retention is the main problem. Please be prepared to ask all questions that are of interest to you and your child before treatment begins.

Two types of treatment are used for soiling with constipation, and they are often combined because they complement one another:
1. Laxatives
2. Toilet training

Many studies have shown that only giving laxatives is not successful. But toilet training alone will not be able to evacuate large amounts of stool. Also, toilet training by itself will not prevent the re-accumulating of stool at a later point. Therefore, the combination of the two is often needed.

In addition to these two important steps, it is important to check the drinking behavior of your child. Some children drink far too little, sometimes only 1.5–2.5 cups ($\approx$ 400–600 ml) per day. Since many parents are not aware of this, the 48-Hour Toilet Chart in Appendix 2 will help you find out what the drinking behavior of your child really is. One quart (≈1 liter) is the absolute minimum a child needs per day; 1.5–2 quarts (≈1.5–2 liters) are desirable, especially if your child is physically active and plays sports. Stool can become softer through increased liquid supply. Also, most laxatives require water to be effective. If your child does not drink enough, make sure to increase the liquid intake of your child and document it in the Drinking Chart in Appendix 3. Either you or the child can complete the chart.

Changes in your child's diet may only be necessary if he or she is a picky eater, i.e., prefers low-fiber foods, such as cookies, white bread, milk, and chocolate. If your child's diet is varied and balanced, there is no need for major changes or food supplements. Studies have shown that increasing fiber alone will not suffice to treat constipation.

2.4 When are laxatives necessary?

If your child's constipation has been going on for a long period of time and has become chronic, treatment without laxatives will not be successful. Laxative treatment consists of two steps:
1. Initial removal of stool called *disimpaction* (see Chapter 2.5).
2. Long-term maintenance treatment with the aim to avoid re-accumulation of stool (see Chapter 2.6).

These steps will be described in the next two chapters.

2.5 How is disimpaction performed?

The initial emptying of the colon is absolutely necessary. If your child has accumulated stool over a long time, it will have formed lumps or even rocks, which can remain there for months and years. The colon can only return to its natural size when the hard, old stool is removed. Therefore, it is important that you do not skip this first step even though it is an unpleasant procedure.

It is important to explain to your child beforehand what will happen during disimpaction as it may be painful when the hard, large lumps of stool are removed or passed. Also, the amount of stool may be so large that it blocks the toilet. Unfortunately, there is no way to avoid this step. When the stool has been removed, your child will feel better immediately. Belly aches, the feeling of pressure, and bloating will become less.

Nowadays, disimpaction with the help of oral laxatives is the preferred method for most children. The medication of choice is polyethylene glycol or PEG, also called macrogol. PEG is available over-the-counter in the United States and can be prescribed in most other countries. PEG consists of a long molecule that stays in the intestines and absorbs water. By binding water, PEG softens the stool and activates the bowel movement. PEG can only work properly when sufficient amounts of liquid are present in the colon. Therefore, it is very important to make sure that your child drinks enough before and during treatment with PEG.

PEG is usually sold as a powder in individual sachets. Liquid forms are sometimes also available. You can dissolve it in water, juice, or other liquids or you can mix it into food such as yoghurt or pudding. The flavor is usually neutral and most children tolerate it. Flavored PEG (chocolate or fruit flavor) is available in some countries. There are very few side effects. However, when the dosage is too high, diarrhea may develop. This can be counteracted by decreasing the dosage.

Large amounts of PEG are needed for disimpaction. Two different treatment strategies are possible:
1. Start with a high dose and maintain it until a large amount of stool has been passed. Then reduce the medication to the amount needed for the maintenance phase. As a general rule, 1.5 g of PEG per kilogram of body weight are required per day and are given in two doses. After stool is passed, the dosage is reduced to approximately 0.4 g of PEG per kilogram body weight per day, given in two doses. Your physician will tell you the exact dosage for your child.
2. The second option is to start with a low or medium dosage and increase it day by day until the colon is empty. If you choose this method, your doctor will tell you exactly how to proceed.

After disimpaction, your physician can check by ultrasound whether the rectum is still enlarged and whether all the stool has been removed. Sometimes it is necessary to repeat the process.

In cases with severe constipation, disimpaction with the help of laxatives may not be enough. Rectal enemas are used instead to help empty the bowels. An enema consists of a plastic bag with fluid (usually sodium phosphate solution) and a tube that is inserted into the anus. For young children, enemas containing sorbitol are preferred as regular enemas might have side effects.

Since children are usually more afraid of enemas than of taking laxatives, it is important that you or the physician explain the process well beforehand. Show your child the tube of the enema and explain that it is much smaller than a thermometer or the stool they pass every day. When the enema is given, the child should lie on his or her side pulling up their legs. The tube of the enema can be lubricated with a cream or a gel to reduce possible irritation. Toddlers and preschool children receive approximately half of the fluid in an enema, school-age children three quarters, and older children all of it. After the liquid has been squeezed into the rectum, the tube is removed. The child should press the buttocks together so that the liquid can remain in the bowel for about 15–20 minutes before going to the toilet. The longer the fluid remains in the bowel, the more thorough the result will be. It is important, however, that the child passes stool and does not retain the enema fluid.

Again, with ultrasound your doctor can easily check whether the colon has been emptied or whether additional enemas are needed. For some children the process may need to be repeated to complete disimpaction. Your doctor will prescribe the type of enema, the required amount of fluid, the number of applications, etc.

In very rare cases, after many years of stool retention, neither oral nor rectal disimpaction is successful. It may be so difficult to remove the old stool that the colon needs to be irrigated. In even more extreme cases, stool has to be removed surgically. Fortunately, these kinds of interventions are very rarely needed. Should they be necessary for your child, be sure that they are performed only by a pediatric specialist in a hospital or in a children's practice.

No matter how disimpaction is achieved, it is a requirement for the successful treatment of your child's incontinence. The old stool simply has to go before your child can take the next steps toward long-term, independent continence.

2.6 What happens during the maintenance phase?

Once the stool has been removed, it is important to prevent the accumulation of new stool. After disimpaction, the colon is still enlarged and all too ready to again accommodate large amounts of stool. The colon needs time to regain its original size and to function normally again. The two most important treatment strategies during this time are oral laxatives and toilet training. This stage of treatment is called the *maintenance phase*. The aim is to maintain what has been achieved: a normal-sized colon without constipation.

Again, the medication of choice is polyethylene glycol (PEG), which has revolutionized the treatment of constipation. PEG is sold over-the-counter in the United States. In many European countries it is approved for the treatment of constipation for toddlers as young as two years old. It is tolerated extremely well and has practically no side effects.

Your physician will determine the dosage of PEG based on how it affects your child. One usually starts with the low dosage of 0.4 g per kilogram of body weight per day, given in two doses. If your child weighs 25 kg, for example, the dosage would be 10 g per day (5 g in the morning and 5 g in the evening). PEG is usually available as a powder and sometimes as a fluid. You can mix it with juice or water or into soft food, such as pudding or apple sauce. Since PEG has a neutral flavor, children usually accept it without problems. If your child insists on a flavored type of PEG, available in some countries, don't hesitate to give it to them. Remember that sufficient fluid intake is vital for PEG to work properly.

If this initial dosage leads to a soft, sausage-like stool, then it can be continued at this level. Please check the Bristol Stool Form Scale as this can be helpful for properly dosing PEG (see Figure 2). If the stool is too soft or even watery, the dosage has to be reduced. If the stool is too hard, medication has to be increased step-by-step until a soft consistency is achieved. The optimal dosage varies greatly from to child to child. Studies suggest that dosages between 0.2 g and 1.5 g per kilogram body weight per day are effective. You should not worry about the dosage, only the consistency of the stool is important. Please talk to your doctor about the dosage required for your child.

PEG can be given over a long period of time. Long-term side effects are not known. It is important, however, that it is given regularly over a sufficiently long period of time. If it has taken months or years for chronic constipation to develop, it will take a comparable time to resolve. It takes time for the colon to shrink back to its original size and to function normally again. Some guidelines recommend that treatment should last between 6 and 24 months. Even when your child has become completely continent, it is advisable to continue with laxatives to prevent a constipation relapse. When PEG is to be discontinued, reduce the dosage slowly and step by step. This way one can monitor whether the constipation has been treated successfully or whether there is still a risk of relapse. If the child has a relapse, the dosage of PEG can be increased again. PEG can be given for as long as it is needed. Some children have taken it for many years, at the end of which normal bowel function was restored and no side effects were reported.

PEG is the laxative of choice and we recommend it wholeheartedly. However, if you prefer a different laxative, lactulose would be an alternative. It is also available as a powder or liquid. Lactulose is a sugar that cannot be absorbed by the body. It binds water in the colon, softening the stool. The dosage again depends on the effect it has on your child and must be adjusted accordingly. If diarrhea or bloating develops, the dosage has to be reduced. Lactulose is less effective than PEG and has more side effects.

In some countries, laxatives such as milk of magnesia or paraffin oil are prescribed. These should not be used as first-line laxatives as they are less effective and have more side effects.

2.7 What is toilet training?

Many studies have shown that toilet training is the most important component of the treatment of soiling (with or without constipation). Toilet training can only work if it is done regularly and the results are documented. Use the charts in the appendix for this purpose. The toilet training chart in Appendix 4 is to be filled out by parents. The version for children is in Appendix 5. Please make sure to fill out the parent chart while your child is doing toilet training.

Toilet training is continued for weeks, months, sometimes even years in combination with laxatives. Even when your child has become continent, it is a good idea to continue the toilet sessions for a while. Your physician or therapist will advise you on the exact length. Toilet training itself has no side effects. Your child's cooperation and the regularity of the training are important.

The principle of toilet training is very simple. After the three main mealtimes of the day (breakfast, lunch, dinner) ask your child to sit on the toilet for 5–10 minutes. The time after a meal is the best for toilet training because the bowels are ready to pass their contents. Hormones and the nervous system of the intestines activate the emptying reflex. Therefore, it is highly important to do the toilet training after mealtimes and not before.

It is important that your child is relaxed while sitting on the toilet and feels safe. If your child is worried about falling in, use a small seat that you place on top of the toilet. You can tell that your child is worried by observing his or her behavior. If they wobble back and forth or cling to the toilet seat, get a small seat to help your child relax.

Another important point is that your child's feet should have contact with the floor. If your child does not reach the ground, place a footrest in front of the toilet. So-called potty trainers or toilet trainer seats combine a small toilet seat with a ladder with handles to hold onto. They allow children to reach the toilet and to use it comfortably.

You should also pay attention to the posture of your child while he or she is sitting on the toilet. They should sit upright with their legs relaxed so that they fall slightly away from each other. Toilet training should be a positive experience. Allow your child to do whatever he or she likes while sitting down. That means that your child can read, draw, sing, play music or other games, listen to stories and fairytales – there is no limit to possible activities. Even reading to your child during the sessions on the toilet is perfectly fine.

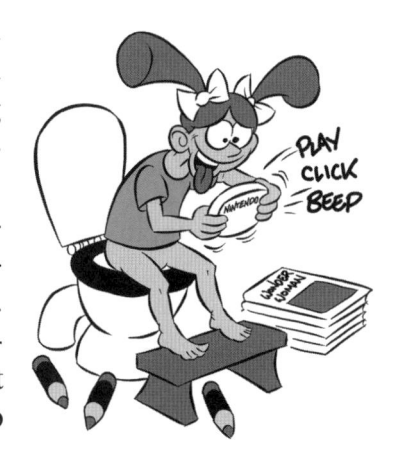

If your child does need a special incentive to go and sit on the toilet, try using toys that are reserved especially for the toilet sessions. Also, coloring books for coloring only during toilet training can be very motivating. It is important that these special toys and books are not available at other times so that they do not lose their appeal and remain incentives for your child. One idea of a mother who came to our practice was a great success! She restricted the playing of computer games to the time of the toilet sessions. Her child was more than willing to go to the toilet and participate in the training. Also, allowing the child to play with the parent's iPad during toilet sessions can be very effective. However, doing this you might find it difficult to get your child off the toilet!

If children like it, toilet sessions can be up to 20 minutes long. However, longer sessions playing computer games are not helpful. Please keep in mind that it is not necessary that your child passes urine or feces during toilet training. It is fine for them to just sit on the toilet after mealtimes. Regular training will help regulate the emptying reflex of the colon and will develop a habit, increasing the likelihood that your child will move his or her bowels after mealtimes. The intention of toilet training is to train this daily habit, thus contributing to both the physical and emotional well-being of your child.

When doing toilet training, be sure to document it on the parent chart in Appendix 4. Seeing the positive changes over time will be very encouraging to you and your child. Note down after each mealtime whether you had to send your child to the toilet or whether he or she went alone. It doesn't matter if you had to send your child – the main point is that the toilet training is done. Going to the toilet alone may be an indication that your child is taking on more responsibility for getting continent. Next, write down whether your child's clothes were wet or dry and whether he or she soiled small or large amounts in the course of the morning/afternoon/evening. Finally, note down whether your child passed urine and/or stool during the sessions. As mentioned before, this is not necessary but may be a sign that things are going well.

Having your child document the training on his or her own chart (see Appendix 5) can be highly motivating! The three columns on the right stand for the mealtimes breakfast, lunch, and dinner. After sitting on the toilet for 5–10 minutes, he or she may draw a symbol into the chart or use a sticker. If additional incentives for cooperation are needed, use rewards for your child. For example, give your child a piece of candy or a sticker for each successful toilet training. For older children, a larger reward at the end of the week may be motivating. Another option is to give your child a small material reward (e.g., a toy car) or a nonmaterial reward (e.g., a visit to the swimming pool or trip to the ice cream parlor) when your child has completed 18 of 21 toilet trainings in a week successfully. Make sure to count the number of sucessful sessions your child had per week. If your child does not fulfill the agreement, e.g., does not reach the agreed upon number of points, he or she does not receive a reward. It is important that the points are not transferred from one week to the next. That means that each week there is a new chance for a reward!

The toilet charts may also be very helpful to your doctor or therapist. They show objectively whether things are going well or whether there is a risk of relapse. Regular visits to your doctor or therapist, for example once a month, are recommended during treatment. If you have questions in between visits, feel free to call the office and to discuss problems right away instead of waiting until your next appointment. Often small changes can increase the motivation of your child. Staying motivated is essential because toilet training can continue for an extended period of time, such as weeks, months, or even years. Even when your child has become continent, it can be helpful to continue filling out the charts. Only when soiling and constipation are over and bowel movements have become regular, can the charts be slowly discontinued. It might also be helpful to keep up the doctor's visits at longer intervals to prevent possible relapses (so-called booster sessions).

The effort you put into toilet training is always worthwhile. When your child is continent, he or she will feel much better as will the other family members.

2.8 What to do if treatment fails?

Despite best efforts and optimal care, some children have difficulty becoming continent. Because standard treatment is not enough for these children, special training programs have been developed (for example, *Urinary and fecal incontinence: A training program for children and adolescents*, Hogrefe Publishing, 2015). This kind of training can be administered to groups of 2–6 children of the same age and gender, or it can be used with individual children. These training programs give information on the digestive tract, nutrition, drinking habits, and toileting behavior. They also feature relaxation techniques, stress management, and cognitive behavioral therapy.

New studies have shown that this kind of training is highly effective because it reduces both incontinence incidents and emotional and behavioral problems. Another advantage is that the treatment is offered on an outpatient basis, which means children can live at home, attend school, and go to the office or clinic for treatment.

2.9 What can I do if my child has special needs?

Children with special needs require additional educational, medical, and psychological assistance. These children may have neurodevelopmental disorders, such as attention-deficit hyperactivity disorder (ADHD) or autism spectrum disorder (ASD), or they may have an intellectual disability or other developmental problems.

Many studies have shown that children with special needs are more often affected by all types of soiling and wetting than children with typical development. Unfortunately, many children with special needs do not receive the required quality of care because wetting and soiling are sometimes seen as part of the disability. They are taken care of by having the children wear diapers instead of assessing and treating the incontinence problem.

The good news is that the assessment and treatment outlined in this book can be applied to children with special needs as well. However, treatment should be adapted to the cognitive level of the child and behavioral problems that might be present need to be taken into account. Sometimes specialized care provided by experts is needed.

If your child has special needs, he or she has the same right to become continent and to stop soiling. Please look for professionals and/or institutions that can help you achieve this goal. Any effort is worthwhile because your child and your family will be much happier once the soiling has stopped.

3 Soiling Without Constipation

3.1 What is soiling without constipation?

As the name implies, some children soil without any signs of constipation. In other words, they go to the toilet every day and pass well-formed stool. They do not experience pain during bowel movements, rarely have abdominal pain (tummy aches), and usually have normal appetite. When these children are examined, their abdomen is soft and no stool can be felt. An ultrasound examination shows that the rectum has a diameter of less than 30 mm (≈ 1 inch).

For this type of soiling the same definition as the one mentioned for soiling with constipation applies. Soiling is considered a disorder when the child soils once a month for the duration of at least three months with other medical causes being excluded. The amount of soiled feces is not relevant – even smearing could be considered soiling. The aim of treatment is complete continence – and not just the reduction of soiling incidents or soiled amounts.

The causes of soiling without constipation are less known. Genetic factors play a less important role than they do for constipation. Soiling without constipation usually does not run in families. Also, typical triggers are not always identifiable.

In the past, experts believed that soiling without constipation was a purely psychological problem. New studies have shown conclusively that this is not the case. The rate of co-occurring psychological symptoms and disorders is just a little bit higher in children who soil without constipation than in children who soil with constipation. This means that the belief that soiling without constipation has psychological causes whereas soiling with constipation has medical causes does not hold true.

Unfortunately, no clear, unambiguous explanation for the development of soiling without constipation is available at the moment. Further studies are needed to answer the many open questions. However, this is not relevant for us because simple and successful treatment exists.

3.2 How do you treat soiling without constipation?

The treatment of soiling without constipation is simple and effective. It is treated with regular toilet training as is soiling with constipation. See Chapter 2.7 for a description of this training and the accompanying charts (Appendix 4 and Appendix 5). Again, it is important to continue the training for long enough to prevent a relapse. Even after the child has become continent, toilet training should be continued for at least some time to stabilize the achievements. Regular visits to your doctor or therapist, for example once a month, are recommended during treatment. Even after the treatment has been completed, booster sessions are a good idea for relapse prevention.

Medication is not needed if your child soils without constipation. Laxatives are not necessary and induce watery and liquid stool, thereby increasing the likelihood of soiling.

This shows again how important it is to clarify right at the beginning of treatment whether the child is constipated or not. If constipation is a problem, then laxatives are necessary for the initial disimpaction and during maintenance therapy. If the child is not constipated, laxatives are absolutely not indicated and should be discontinued if they are being taken.

4 Toilet Refusal

The typical behavior of toilet refusal is well known to many parents. The toilet is used for passing urine without any problems, but not for moving the bowels. Children insist on a diaper for this purpose and do not use the toilet. This behavior is very common in toddlers if it is just temporary. Toilet refusal syndrome as a condition is present when this behavior is maintained for more than one month continuously.

4.1 How does toilet refusal develop?

The reasons why some children refuse to go to the toilet are not quite clear. It seems to be a common but temporary phenomenon in many toddlers. This behavior is completely harmless and without long-term consequences if it is not continued over a longer period of time, i.e., for longer than 3–4 months.

Some children who refuse to use the toilet to move their bowels have additional risk factors, such as stressful life events and behavioral problems and disorders. Some children show oppositional behavior, argue a lot, and break rules. They can be agitated, irritable, and angry, showing verbal aggression, and having temper tantrums. In addition, some children are anxious or show signs of sibling rivalry.

Studies have shown that late potty training and a laissez-faire attitude of parents can be associated with toilet refusal. The risk of toilet refusal and constipation increases when potty training is started when the child is 42 months or older.

Constipation and toilet refusal are closely related. Studies have shown that a pre-existing constipation can increase the risk of toilet refusal. In these cases, the children have constipation first and then develop the habit of passing feces only into diapers, sometimes because of fear of painful bowel movements. This habit then is maintained and over time becomes chronic. Other children develop toilet refusal first and then become constipated. When they do not get the diaper as desired, they hold back the stool until chronic constipation has developed. Irrespective of the starting point, long-term toilet refusal can lead to severe constipation with enlarged colon and rectum. This development is to be avoided because the treatment of toilet refusal combined with constipation is more difficult.

4.2　How do you treat toilet refusal?

Treatment is different for temporary toilet refusal in toddlers and young children compared to chronic toilet refusal in older preschoolers and school-age children.

Temporary toilet refusal fortunately happens for just a short time and has no negative long-term consequences. Many parents are worried about this peculiar behavior of their children, i.e., insisting on a diaper to pass feces, and try to break the habit. Because children can be very stubborn, parents sometimes give the diaper and at other times insist that the potty or the toilet is used. This lack of consequence often reinforces toilet refusal. The child obstinately insists on the diaper and rather holds back stool than to submit to the pressure of the parents. Very often this interplay leads to arguments, verbal aggression, and tantrums with emotions running high.

Treating temporary toilet refusal is relatively easy. The main goal is to reduce the stress and pressure the family experiences. Have your child wear the diaper all the time, not only when he or she wants to move their bowls. Explain that the diaper stays on until he or she is ready to go to the toilet.

To further reduce stress, stop potty training for the time being. This break can be a great relief for the entire family. Plan trips and fun activities for the whole family to strengthen the positive aspects of your parent–child relationship. Also, engage in regular play times with your child, e.g., 10 minutes per day. Allow the child to choose the game you'll be playing during these sessions and make sure that you are fully present and not distracted by other activities or chores. Additional therapy is usually

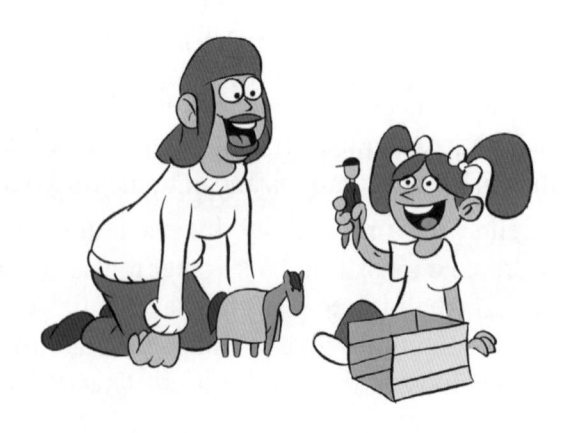

4. Toilet Refusal

not necessary. When the time has come, your child will go to the toilet and give up the diaper voluntarily.

For children with **chronic toilet refusal,** this approach will not have the desired effect. Have your child wear a diaper all day and not just on demand, and start toilet training as described in Chapter 2.7. Ask your child to sit on the toilet for 5–10 minutes after the main meals, i.e., three times a day. This combined approach reduces stress and anger because it eliminates the fights over the diaper and restricts potty training to the times after meals. The toilet training will train the emptying reflexes of the colon the same way as in children with constipation.

If your child has retained large amounts of stool because of chronic toilet refusal, then the same laxative treatment is needed as for children with constipation. If necessary, disimpaction with the laxative polyethylene glycol (PEG) is done first, followed by a lower dosage for maintenance over a longer period of time (see Chapter 2.4 and Chapter 2.5).

Because chronic toilet refusal has a higher rate of accompanying psychological problems and disorders than temporary toilet refusal, child psychological/psychiatric assessment may be needed as well as counseling. Additional mental healthcare can further reduce stress and minimize difficulties in social situations and at home for your child.

5 Soiling With Wetting

In addition to soiling, does your child sometimes wet his or her pants or the bed? If that is so, then your child has what is called a *combined incontinence* problem, which is quite common. Some children with soiling also wet during the day and during the night.

5.1 How does soiling with wetting develop?

It may be a great relief for parents to know that the combination of soiling and wetting is very common. If a child retains stool, it is very likely that he or she also holds back urine as the pelvic floor is one functional unit. If urine is retained, the likelihood for urinary tract infections and for wetting increases.

In addition, the retained stool in constipation can impede the function of the bladder because the colon presses against the bladder and induces contractions. This is felt as an urge to empty the bladder and can lead to daytime wetting. Retention of stool can also have a negative effect on the emptying of the bladder so that the urine flow is interrupted and the child has to strain. Finally, both colon and bladder function are coordinated by the same centers in the brain so that a disorder of one system can compromise the other.

It is often not possible to identify the exact cause(s) for combined soiling and wetting, and it is not necessary to do so for treatment. Thorough assessment and the clear diagnosis of the type of soiling and the type of wetting are what counts. If you would like further information on wetting, please consult our companion guide *Wetting in children and adolescents: A practical guide for parents, teachers, and caregivers* (Hogrefe Publishing, 2017).

5.2 What is the definition of daytime wetting?

Daytime wetting is called *nonorganic (or functional) urinary incontinence* and is an involuntary and intermittent wetting. It is considered a disorder when the child is older than 5 years, the wetting persists for three months at a frequency of at least once a month, and if medical causes and complications have been excluded. As you can see, the definitions of soiling and wetting are quite similar except for the age definition. Wetting is so common among four-year-old children that it is considered part of normal development and maturation. Only if it persists after the child is five years old, it is considered to be a condition.

Daytime wetting is a disorder of the bladder function. Different types of daytime wetting exist. The three most common types are called *urge incontinence*, *voiding postponement,* and *dysfunctional voiding*. This might be confusing at the first, but the three types are easily differentiated.

Urge incontinence is an inborn disorder that causes the bladder to contract spontaneously and repeatedly during filling. The brain does not sufficiently suppress these contractions. They are perceived as an urge to go to the toilet, which is the reason why the term urge incontinence has been adopted. It is typical for children with this type of incontinence that they run to the toilet suddenly many times during the day. They pass only small amounts of urine every time. Their clothing is often damp because small amounts of urine are lost throughout the day. Many children use holding maneuvers to stop the urge, such as pressing the thighs together.

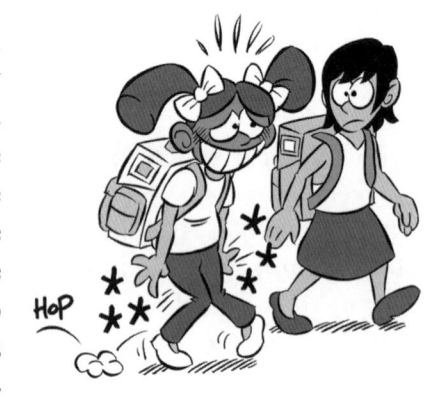

In contrast, children with **voiding postponement** rarely go to the toilet and then void large volumes of urine. Even though they have to go to the toilet, they hold back the urine with holding maneuvers. This postponement slowly turns into a chronic habit and is maintained over time. Voiding postponement is an acquired disorder that is often accompanied by oppositional defiant disorder.

The third common type, **voiding dysfunction**, is a problem with the emptying of the bladder. Instead of relaxing, the closing muscle (sphincter) of the bladder contracts so that the urine flow is interrupted. Typical signs are straining at the beginning and during voiding and an interrupted stream. With dysfunctional voiding, urinary tract infections and other medical complications are common and have to be identified and treated.

5.3 What is bedwetting?

Bedwetting is officially called *nocturnal enuresis*, or enuresis for short, and is an intermittent wetting during sleep. It is considered a disorder when it persists for 3 months with a minimum frequency of one incident of bedwetting per month, when the child is 5 years and older, and when medical causes and complications have been excluded. Again, the age definition is different from soiling because bedwetting is common in four-year-old children.

Four different forms of enuresis can be differentiated. *Primary bedwetting* means that the child has never been dry. *Secondary bedwetting* means that he or she had a relapse after a dry period of at least six months. If a child wets during sleep but has normal bladder function, the disorder is called *monosymptomatic bedwetting* or *simple bedwetting*. If there is a bladder dysfunction, the term *non-monosymptomatic bedwetting* is used. This may be a bit confusing, but the diagnosis is very important for treatment. You will find more details on wetting in the companion guide.

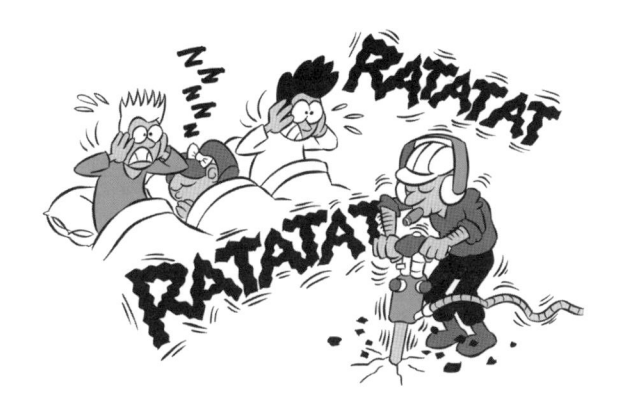

Nocturnal enuresis is a genetic maturational disorder of the central nervous system, i.e., the brain, and not a disorder of the bladder. Three factors are important for why bedwetting happens: (1) some children produce too much urine at night, (2) other children sleep very deeply and have difficulty waking up, and (3) in some children the brain does not suppress the emptying reflex of the bladder during sleep.

5.4 How is wetting assessed?

Again, you will find detailed information in the companion guide on wetting. The first step in the assessment of bedwetting is the physical examination of the child. This should include a urinalysis to exclude urinary tract infections. Questionnaires and charts also provide helpful information. If your child wets, fill out the 48-Hour Toilet Chart (see Appendix 2), making sure to measure the amounts of urine as this will provide important information for correct diagnosis.

The diagnosis of the type of wetting is the prerequisite for optimal treatment. In principle, every type of wetting has to be treated separately and specifically.

5.5 How do you treat daytime wetting?

Because of space constraints, the treatment of wetting is not presented here in full detail. Please see the companion guide for further information. The most important aspects of treatment are summarized here to give you an orientation.

If your child has **urge incontinence**, i.e., if he or she often feels the need to urinate and goes to the toilet but voids only small amounts of urine, then different types of charts are helpful for keeping track and motivating your child. Documentation is also important to focus the attention on voiding habits and to see changes throughout treatment. Ask your child not to use holding maneuvers but to go to the toilet right away when he or she feels the urge to urinate. If he or she gets to the toilet in time without wetting the pants, have him or her draw a flag (or some other symbol) into the chart. If the pants do get wet, ask him or her draw a cloud or some other symbol. Of course, your child can use any symbol he or she likes as long as the wet and dry times can be kept apart. It may be that your child goes to the toilet 10 times or more per day at the beginning of treatment. In the course of therapy, the number of dry toilet times (flags) will become fewer as the number of times your child goes to the toilet normalizes. The the number of wetting incidences (clouds) should become fewer as well. Filling in charts is enough motivation for about one third of the children to get dry. About two thirds of the children need additional medication such as oxybutynin and propiverine. The function of these medications is simple: They "quiet down" the bladder so that it can hold more urine and reduce the spontaneous contractions, relieving urinary urgency. If medication is needed, the training of focusing on the urge, going to the toilet right away without holding maneuvers, and continuing documentation in charts should be carried out as before.

Children with **voiding postponement** rarely go to the toilet and postpone emptying their bladder. The aim of treatment is to increase the number of visits to the toilet per day. This is called *timed voiding*. The children are asked to go to the toilet at least seven times per day. Every time they urinate, they note this down in a chart. If they wet during the day, they should note this down as well. By increasing the times the child urinates per day, this type of daytime wetting usually stops.

Children with **voiding dysfunction** do not relax the pelvic floor while urinating. The closing muscle of the bladder does not open but contracts instead. This disorder is best treated with biofeedback training because it allows the children to become aware of what is happening in their bodies while they are trying to void and then to learn how to control it. The contraction of the pelvic floor is presented either acoustically or visually with child-friendly animations. The training can be carried out at home but is most often offered at specialized centers.

Many parents ask what toilet habits are considered normal. For orientation the following numbers might help:
- Normally, children go to the toilet 5–7 times a day to urinate. In children with urge incontinence, this is often increased to 8 or more times; in those with voiding postponement it is decreased to 4 times or fewer.
- The maximum volume of urine considered normal is calculated easily: Add 1 to the age of your child and multiply it by 30 ml. For example, if your child is six years old, multiply 7 by 30. This gives you 210 ml (≈ 7 fl. oz), which is the approximate maximum amount of urine your child produces per day. In children with urge incontinence, this volume is reduced to 30–80 ml (≈ 1–3 fl. oz); in children with voiding postponement it can be greatly increased.

- Straining and an interrupted urine stream, as is typical in children with voiding dysfunction, are not normal and should be examined and treated.

5.6 How do you treat bedwetting?

Again, only the basic principles can be dealt with here. It is a good idea to start treatment by asking your child to fill out a chart (see the companion guide on wetting). Children mark dry nights with a sun and wet nights with a cloud. Of course, other symbols can be used as well. Simply by documenting the wet and dry nights, approximately 15% of children with bedwetting become dry without further treatment. For the remaining 85% of children, other treatment steps are necessary.

The treatment of choice is *alarm treatment*. Many studies have shown that this is by far the most effective form of therapy for bedwetting. Approximately 70% of children achieve dryness and remain continent. No other form of treatment has a comparable success rate. The prerequisite for alarm treatment is that children and parents are motivated and willing to conduct alarm treatment for up to 16 weeks.

The bedwetting alarm consists of a moisture sensor and a bell, connected by a wire. There are two types of alarms. The body-worn alarm has a sensor that is placed in the underpants and a bell that is attached to the pajamas close to the ear of the child. Nowadays, child-friendly alarms are available. The bedside alarm consists of a mat that is put under the bed sheet and a bell that is placed next to the bed. Both types of alarms work the same way – they go off as soon as the sensor detects moisture. The children should be allowed to choose the one they prefer.

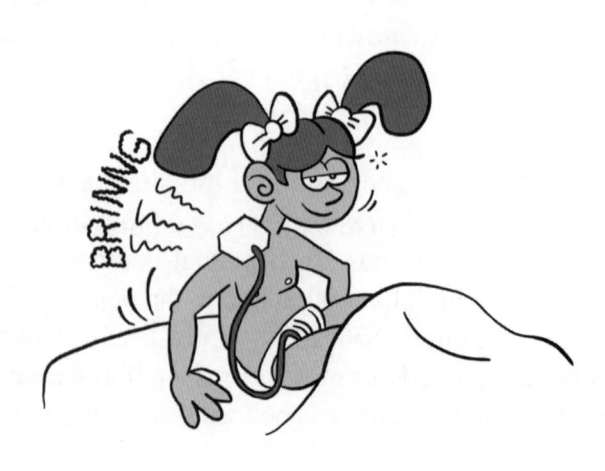

The sensor is put in place at bedtime and switched on. After a dry night, no other interventions are necessary and the alarm can be switched off the next morning. If bedwetting does happen, it is important that your child wakes up and goes quickly to the toilet to pass the remaining urine. After the pajamas and sheets have been changed, put the sensor back in place and switch the alarm on again. Older children might do all this on their own but young children will need the help of their parents. Document the alarm treatment in a special chart and bring it to the appointments with your doctor or therapist. The exact mechanisms how the bedwetting alarm works are not known, but many studies have shown conclusively that it is highly effective. Approximately two thirds of the children learn to sleep through the night with a full bladder. One third of the children learn to wake up when the bladder is full and go to the toilet. It is not of importance how treatment success is achieved, the main point is that your child gets dry. After 14 dry nights in a row, the alarm treatment can be discontinued.

Some children reach dryness quickly, for example, after 6–8 weeks of alarm treatment. Other children need more time. When alarm treatment continues over several weeks, the motivation of your child to actively participate might become less. If this happens, combine the alarm treatment with little rewards. It is important that the child is not rewarded for dry nights but exclusively for his or her cooperation, over which the child has direct control. If alarm treatment is not successful after 16 weeks, it is recommended to take a break from it.

Another type of treatment is *medication with desmopressin*, a drug that reduces the urine production during sleep. Approximately 70% of children either stop bedwetting or have fewer wet nights. However, most children encounter a relapse when the medication is discontinued. The long-term effects are less favorable than the ones for alarm treatment by which at least 50% of children achieve permanent long-term dryness. Desmopressin is especially indicated:
- for children who are not motivated for alarm treatment,
- when the parents have other obligations or cannot guarantee support for their child for several weeks,
- for children who have to gain dryness quickly, for example, prior to vacations or school trips,
- when alarm treatment has failed.

Desmopressin is well tolerated. It is given in the evening as a regular tablet (0.2 mg to 0.4 mg) or as a melt tablet

(120 µg to 240 µg). If the medication does not work after four weeks, it should be discontinued as the child might be a nonresponder. Slight abdominal pain and headaches are known side effects of the drug. The only serious side effect occurs rarely and when children drink too much liquid after taking the drug or take too high a dose of the medication. Desmopressin may lead to a dilution of the blood and the reduction of sodium concentration, which can cause fainting and unconsciousness. Therefore, it is recommended not to drink anything after taking the medication in the evening.

5.7 How do you treat combined soiling and wetting?

There is a recommended treatment sequence that should be followed.

Soiling with or without constipation is always treated first. The treatment of soiling may have the positive effect that children stop wetting and do not need further therapy. Also, the risk for developing urinary tract infections is reduced.

If your child continues to wet after he or she has stopped soiling, daytime wetting should be treated before bedwetting. When the type of daytime wetting has been assessed and diagnosed (urge incontinence, postponement, dysfunctional voiding, etc.), it is treated according to the methods described in Chapter 5.5. Since daytime wetting is always a dysfunction of the bladder, the treatment of this dysfunction will stop bedwetting in many children.

5. Soiling With Wetting

If your child no longer soils and has stopped wetting during the day but continues to wet his or her bed at night, then bedwetting should be treated last. The treatment of choice is alarm treatment as described in Chapter 5.6. If this is not possible or has failed, the second choice is treatment with desmopressin.

6 Soiling and Psychological Problems

6.1 How common are psychological problems and disorders in children who soil?

Many studies have shown conclusively that approximately 30–50% of all children with soiling have additional, clinically relevant psychological disorders. This rate is much higher than in children with wetting. Therefore, screening for psychological problems with a broadband questionnaire, such as the Child Behavior Checklist (CBCL) or the Strengths and Difficulties Questionnaire (SDQ), is always recommended. If a disorder is suspected, more detailed child psychological or psychiatric assessment is needed.

There are no psychological disorders that are typically associated with soiling. Studies have shown that some children suffer from so-called *internalizing disorders*. Internalizing means that the psychological symptoms are mainly directed inwardly. Children with depression, for example, are unhappy, sad, pessimistic, have fewer interests, and are involved in fewer activities. Children with an anxiety disorder can have phobias of animals or other objects, they can show separation anxiety or anxiety in social contacts, or they worry a lot without apparent reason.

Children who soil can also have so-called *externalizing disorders* with outwardly observable behavioral problems. A common disorder of this type is attention-deficit/hyperactivity disorder (ADHD). Children with ADHD are hyperactive, always on the run, have a reduced attention span, are easily distracted, or act impulsively. Children with oppositional defiant disorder (ODD) can be angry or irritable, often lose their temper, show argumentative or defiant behavior, and can even be vindictive. Some children suffer from conduct disorder (CD) with antisocial tendencies. For each of these different disorders, specific treatments are available.

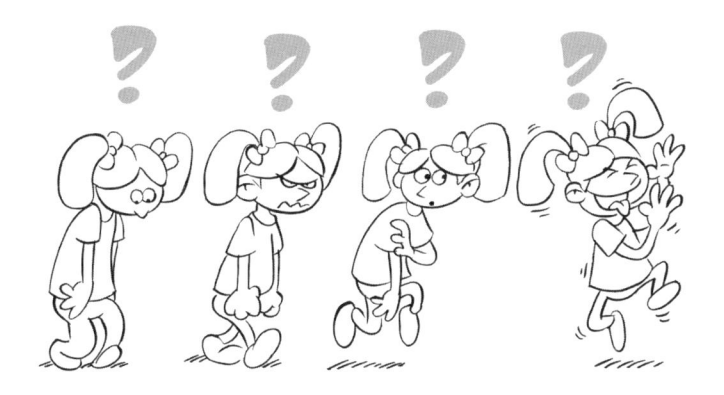

Please keep in mind that most children with soiling, i.e., 50–70%, do not have additional psychological disorders. These children may be unhappy, sad, or distressed as a reaction to the soiling and the many negative social consequences they experience because of that, such as bullying or teasing. These reactions are, of course, not disorders and with successful treatment of the soiling the distress will disappear. Psychotherapies are not necessary in these cases.

6.2 How do you assess psychological disorders?

Again, the first step is conducting a thorough assessment. The diagnosis of a psychological disorder requires experience and training. This can be done by child psychologists, child psychiatrists, and pediatricians with special training. There are clear criteria for the identification of psychological disorders. These criteria are laid down in the *Diagnostic and Statistical Manual of Mental Disorders* (DSM-5) which is used in the United States and many other countries. In other countries of the world, the *International Classification of Diseases* (ICD-10) system, established by the World Health Organization, is used.

Part of a mental healthcare assessment is taking down the detailed history of the current symptoms and the development of the disorder. The behavior of the child is observed and recorded. Behavioral questionnaires are usually completed and, if necessary, an intelligence test and other psychological tests are performed. A physical examination is always done. In many hospitals an EEG (electroencephalogram) is performed. Other examinations are only necessary if they are indicated by the results of the basic assessment.

6.3 How do you treat soiling if psychological problems or disorders are present?

Soiling is always treated according to the principles described above even if a psychological disorder is present. The heart of the treatment is toilet training that may be combined with laxatives if the child suffers from constipation. This basic treatment should always be followed.

If an additional psychological disorder is present, this has to be treated separately. If your child has depression or suffers from an anxiety disorder, psychotherapies can be very effective. Psychotherapy should only be directed at the disorder that has been diagnosed, such as depression or anxiety, and not at the soiling. In many cases, cognitive behavioral therapy (CBT) is the method of choice. It is a type of therapy in which problematic behavior is the focus (the behavioral aspect of therapy) and dysfunctional thoughts are addressed (the cognitive aspect of therapy). In other cases, psychodynamic therapy, which addresses unconscious processes, may be in order. With young children, the medium of psychotherapy is typically play, while older children and adolescents can be treated with verbal psychotherapy. Parental counseling is always part of the therapeutic process.

In some disorders, such as ADHD, medication can be extremely helpful. Studies have shown that stimulant therapy has positive effects on concentration and hyperactivity – and also increases adherence and cooperation with incontinence therapy.

As there are many different therapies available, it is important that you chose the type of therapy that will be most effective for your child and the specific disorder present at the time. A prerequisite for making the right choice is a clear diagnosis. Unnecessary psychotherapies should be avoided.

There are no general recommendations for the sequence of psychotherapies – it is always determined by the needs of your child and your family. In most cases, soiling and any accompanying behavioral disorders can be treated at the same time. If your child, for example, has severe ADHD, it might be better to start with the treatment of that. The reason is that a good treatment with stimulants will make it much easier for your child to follow toilet training and to fill out charts. In other words, the treatment of ADHD can have a positive influence on the soiling treatment. If your child has been diagnosed with a mild anxiety disorder, it might be best to wait with the treatment of that until your child is continent. Many children who have stopped soiling display fewer emotional and behavioral symptoms so that additional therapies might no longer be necessary. In any case, be sure to discuss the treatment and treatment sequence with your therapist or doctor.

6.4 Where can you treat soiling and psychological disorders?

Most children with soiling can be treated as outpatients: They stay at home, go to school, and attend therapy appointments at a clinic or practice. This works very well for most children.

For children with soiling and severe behavioral disorders, professional, intensive treatment in an in-patient setting can be of great help. If the behavioral problems are less marked, day clinics are a good alternative. However, in day-clinic treatment toilet training has to be done both at the clinic and at home. This can be difficult for some children, while others manage it easily.

In summary, most children can be treated as outpatients without any problems. Only with severe psychological disorders should an in-patient setting be considered. Even then, the time spent in in-patient treatment should be kept to a minimum.

7 Concluding Remarks

The aim of this guide was to give you a short overview of the different types of soiling and to inform you about the many available treatments. Soiling is an official disorder according to the World Health Organization. It is a condition that needs to be medically assessed and can be treated with excellent outcomes for many children. You and your child have the right to be treated effectively and professionally.

If your child wants to stop soiling and is distressed, please consult your pediatrician or general practitioner and find the best professional help you can get. In many countries, pediatricians, general practitioners, child psychiatrists, child psychologists, therapists, and other professionals will be able to support you. Never lose sight of the final goal. When your child has reached continence, many other problems will very likely have resolved as well. To reach this goal, it is worthwhile to keep up the effort and give the best you can. I wish you and your child all the best and hope that you will be successful!

Further Reading

Companion guide:
von Gontard, A. (2017). *Wetting in children and adolescents: A practical guide for parents, teachers, and caregivers.* Boston, MA: Hogrefe Publishing. http://doi.org/10.1027/00488-000

Online sources:
International Children's Continence Society (ICCS): http://i-c-c-s.org/parents/
Strengths and Difficulties Questionnaire (SDQ): http://www.sdqinfo.com
von Gontard, A. (2012). Enuresis. In J. Rey (Ed.), *IACAPAP textbook of child and adolescent mental health.* Available at http://iacapap.org/iacapap-textbook-of-child-and-adolescent-mental-health
von Gontard, A. (2012). Encopresis. In J. Rey (Ed.), *IACAPAP textbook of child and adolescent mental health.* Available at http://iacapap.org/iacapap-textbook-of-child-and-adolescent-mental-health

Important ICCS (International Children's Continence Society) documents:
Austin, P. F., Bauer, S., Bower, W., Chase, J., Franco, I., Hoebeke, P., ... Nevéus, T. (2016). The standardization of terminology of bladder function in children and adolescents: Update report from the standardization committee of the International Children's Continence Society (ICCS). *Neurology and Urodynamics, 35*, 471–481. http://doi.org/10.1002/nau.22751
Burgers, R. E., Mugie, S. M., Chase, J., Cooper, C. S., von Gontard, A., Siggaard Rittig, C., ... Benninga, M. (2013). Management of functional constipation in children with lower urinary tract symptoms: Report from the Standardisation Committee of the International Children's Continence Society. *Journal of Urology, 190*, 29–36. http://doi.org/ 10.1016/j.juro.2013.01.001

Koppen, I. J. N., von Gontard, A., Chase, J., Cooper, C. S., Rittig, C. S., Bauer, S. B., ... Benninga, M. A. (2016). Management of functional nonretentive fecal incontinence in children: Recommendations from the International Children's Continence Society. *Journal of Pediatric Urology, 12*, 56–64. Advance online publication. http://doi.org/10.1016/j.jpurol.2015.09.008

von Gontard, A., Baeyens, D., Van Hoecke, E., Warzak, W., & Bachmann, C. (2011). Psychological and psychiatric issues in urinary and fecal incontinence. *Journal of Urology, 185*, 1432–1437. http://doi.org/10.1016/j.juro.2010.11.051

For professionals:

Equit, M., Sambach, H., Niemczyk, J., & von Gontard, A. (2015). *Urinary and fecal incontinence: A training program for children and adolescents*. Boston, MA: Hogrefe Publishing. http://doi.org/10.1027/00460-000

Franco, I., Austin, P., Bauer, S., von Gontard, A., & Homsy, Y. (Eds.). (2015). *Pediatric incontinence: Evaluation and clinical management*. Hoboken, NJ: Wiley-Blackwell.

von Gontard, A., & Neveus, T. (2006). *Management of disorders of bladder and bowel control in childhood*. London, UK: MacKeith Press.

Appendices

Appendix 1   Soiling Questionnaire
Appendix 2   48-Hour Toilet Chart
Appendix 3   Drinking Chart
Appendix 4   Toilet Training Chart for Parents
Appendix 5   Toilet Training Chart for Children

Appendix 1

Soiling Questionnaire

Name _____ Date of birth _____ Date _____

Frequency of soiling

Does your child soil during the day?	☐ yes	☐ no
How often does your child soil during the day?	_____	days per week
	_____	days per month
How often does your child soil per day?	_____	times per day
Does your child soil during the night?	☐ yes	☐ no
How often does your child soil during the night?	_____	nights per week
	_____	nights per month

Soiling symptoms

If your child soils, how large is the amount of stool?	☐ only smearing
	☐ smearing and stool
	☐ only stool
What is the consistency of your child's stool?	☐ hard
	☐ soft
	☐ watery

Relapses

Has your child ever had a period in his or her life without soiling?	☐ yes	☐ no
If yes, at what age did this occur?	From age	_____ (in years or months)
	to age	_____ (in years or months)

Toileting behavior

On how many days per week does your child pass stool into the toilet?	_____ days per week
How many times per day does your child defecate?	_____ times per day

---

This page may be reproduced by the purchaser for personal/professional use.
From A. von Gontard: *Soiling in Children and Adolescents:
A Guide for Parents, Teachers, and Caregivers* © 2017 Hogrefe Publishing

How large is the amount of stool in the toilet?	☐ small
	☐ medium
	☐ large
What is the consistency of your child's stool in the toilet?	☐ hard
	☐ soft
	☐ watery
	☐ with blood
Is defecation painful for your child?	☐ yes ☐ no
Does your child have stomach or abdominal pains?	☐ yes ☐ no

Perception of and reactions to soiling

Does your child suffer emotionally because of the soiling?	☐ yes ☐ no
Is your child motivated for treatment?	☐ yes ☐ no
Have you punished your child because of the soiling?	☐ yes ☐ no

Wetting

How often does your child go to the toilet to urinate?	_____ times per day
Does your child wet during the day?	☐ yes ☐ no
If yes, how often?	_____ days per week
Does your child wet at night?	☐ yes ☐ no
If yes, how often?	_____ days per week
How much fluid does your child drink per day?	_____ cups/liters per day

---

This page may be reproduced by the purchaser for personal/professional use.
From A. von Gontard: *Soiling in Children and Adolescents:
A Guide for Parents, Teachers, and Caregivers* © 2017 Hogrefe Publishing

Appendix 2

48-Hour Toilet Chart						
Name _____ Date of birth _____ Date _____						
Time	Urine on toilet (oz/ml)	Wetting: damp/ wet?	Bowel movement on toilet	Soiling	Fluid intake (oz/ml)	Comments/ observations

This page may be reproduced by the purchaser for personal/professional use.
From A. von Gontard: *Soiling in Children and Adolescents:*
A Guide for Parents, Teachers, and Caregivers © 2017 Hogrefe Publishing

Instructions for 48-Hour Toilet Chart

Dear parents,

This chart is suitable for all children who have combined soiling and wetting. In order to assess and treat the continence problem of your child, it is necessary to observe the toileting behavior of your child. The information gathered in the chart will be very helpful to your doctor or therapist. Please fill out this chart on a day when your child is at home (e.g., weekend or holiday). Note down when your child goes to the toilet and/or any wetting or soiling incidents. Start this on the morning of one day and continue until the next morning. **If possible, fill out the chart for two days in a row (48 hours) – this will provide more reliable information.**

Please talk to your child beforehand about what the chart is for and what you'll be doing with it. Do not send your child to the toilet. Instead, your child should tell you when he/she wants to go to the toilet. Ask your child to empty the urine into a measuring cup. Record the amount of urine in the chart with the time of day before discarding it.

If your child wets his/her clothes, note down the time and whether the clothes were wet or damp.

Please write down when your child goes to the toilet to move his/her bowels. Do the same for any soiling incidents.

If you notice holding maneuvers, i.e., that your child crosses his/her legs or squats, please write this down in the observations/comments column. Feel free to write down anything else relevant that you observe.

Finally, please measure and note down the amount of liquid your child drinks during the day, making sure to record the times as well.

Thank you very much for your help!

This page may be reproduced by the purchaser for personal/professional use.
From A. von Gontard: *Soiling in Children and Adolescents:
A Guide for Parents, Teachers, and Caregivers*   © 2017 Hogrefe Publishing

Appendix 3

	Drinking Chart									

This chart belongs to:
_____

My symbol for drinking:

	1	2	3	4	5	6	7	8	9	10
Monday										
Tuesday										
Wednesday										
Thursday										
Friday										
Saturday										
Sunday										

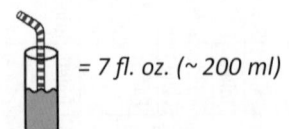

= 7 fl. oz. (~ 200 ml)

Appendix 4

Toilet Training Chart for Parents

Toilet training: 3 times a day for 5–10 minutes after the main meals

Date:		Monday	Tuesday	Wednesday	Thursday	Friday	Saturday	Sunday
Morning	Child sent (→) Child went on his/her own (!)							
	Pants: dry (d) wet (w) Stool amount small (S) Stool amount large (L)							
	Toilet: urine (u) stool (s)							
Midday	Child sent (→) Child went on his/her own (!)							
	Pants: dry (d) wet (w) Stool amount small (S) Stool amount large (L)							
	Toilet: urine (u) stool (s)							
Evening	Child sent (→) Child went on his/her own (!)							
	Pants: dry (d) wet (w) Stool amount small (S) Stool amount large (L)							
	Toilet: urine (u) stool (s)							

This page may be reproduced by the purchaser for personal/professional use.
From A. von Gontard: *Soiling in Children and Adolescents: A Guide for Parents, Teachers, and Caregivers*

© 2017 Hogrefe Publishing

Appendix 5

Toilet Training Chart			
		This chart belongs to: _____	
Monday			
Tuesday			
Wednesday			
Thursday			
Friday			
Saturday			
Sunday			